Thank you so much for reading my book, I truly appreciate it and I hope you enjoy it!

I just wanted to let you know that I'm a parent who spends long hours and lots of time alone in front of a computer writing...

I love it, but sometimes it's...Ugh.

Especially when I would like to spend more time with the family.

So in addition to book writing and publishing, I've also started dabbling in the License Rights business model:

Basically, I recommend high quality information products to folks interested in making extra income...and...

...make a tiny fortune in the process.

I'm biased, but I've found this to be the best one out there, head and shoulders above the rest.

Check it out and let me know what you think

http://www.mylicenserights.com/

Thanks again!

# Table of Contents

## Introduction

*And do not get drunk with wine, for that is debauchery, but be filled with the Spirit - Anonymous*

What you are going to learn here are the benefits of Red wine. But remember that red wine is good when enjoyed in moderation.

What's so great about Red wine you may ask? After all, wine is just fermented fruit juice. In simple terms, fermentation is the conversion of sugar into alcohol with the help of yeast. Wine is made from a number of fruits from apples to pomegranates but here we will talk about Red wine made out of grapes.

Red wine is as old as civilization itself. Grapes used to grow all over the world in the wild, but mainly in Eastern Russia, Iran and Turkey. The oldest-known winery was discovered in Armenia and has been dated back to 4100 BC. There are many myths and legends on Red wine. Wine finds a mention in old biblical writings. Wine has also been used as an excuse by various people and authorities to justify their actions. Greek mythology mentions discovery of wine by Dionysus because of which he became the god of wine.

### History of Red Wine

The discovery of wine in other parts of the world has sometimes been accidental. In Persian legend, King Jamshid banished a lady of his harem. This woman sought out a jar marked "poison" containing the remains of the grapes that were rotten, spoiled and undrinkable. After drinking the fermented wine, she found herself in a different world. She introduced this magical liquid to the king, who soon became captivated by it and took her back. Obviously, since then, wine has been a favorite drink of kings and royalty.

Fast forward to the present, wine making is now an industry. Modern technology has enabled production of massive amount of wine. The consumption has also increased manifold. What used to be an exclusive drink for the upper class is now available to every one of us. In fact, scientific methods of wine production have ensured that everyone has access to quality wines at reasonable rates.

Wine production is not exactly a science, nor an art. It's a subtle mixture of both science and art – very much like the flavor of wine itself. Wine making began in Europe and therefore people from this side of the world tend to give more importance to the artistic part of wine making and consumption. The new world or more specifically the Americans are more adept at using technology to create quality wines. You must remember that wine has different flavor, style, taste and pungency, if you may call it. You can move to a different level of consciousness by simply sipping on wine. Is getting high on spirit the only benefit of Red wine? Or does it have any other beneficial effects?

### Red Wine is Good for Health

Drinking Red wine is great for your health. But remember that everything needs moderation. Too much of a good thing can be a bad thing. This goes for Red wine. This fact is known to all and it has never been a secret. Red wine has been used in religious ceremonies in many cultures. The last supper of Christ describes the consumption of wine in detail. Some experts say that Red wine looks like blood and is therefore used in rituals and religious rites as a substitute.

Red wine is not for special occasions alone. It can be had every day and during every meal. People in certain places in the Mediterranean enjoy their cup of divine bliss all the time. You can drink Red wine alone or with other foodstuff. You can also mix alcohol with wine. In fact modern wines do offer a combination of liquor and wine. Some connoisseurs may find this practice distasteful but there are others who find pure undiluted wine devoid of a good royal kick. It must be understood that wine drinking itself is an art. It has to be done slowly and in a relaxed manner. The spirit creeps in your head slowly and alters your consciousness. Obviously it's not for a person in a hurry.

### Cooking with Red Wine

What kind of food goes best with Red wine? The subject is quite controversial. Some claim that good wine doesn't need support from food. There are those who swear that no food is complete without a good dollop of wine. A party is never complete without the wine flowing. Food acquires a distinct flavor when added with food. Generally Red wine is associated with red meat – mutton, beef and venison. White wine on the other hand is supposed to go well with fish and chicken. To get the best out of your Red wine you must experiment. Individual tastes differ. Even seasons matter where wine is concerned. A salubrious climate can do wonders to your wine experience.

## Red Wine aids Weight Loss

Coming back to the effect of Red wine on health, every known civilization has saluted wine for its beneficial effect. The immediate effect of consuming Red Wine is for relaxation. Your mind and body slowly release the tension making you feel euphoric or calm depending on your mental and physiological makeup. Remember that we are talking of moderate consumption. Make no mistake that you can get drunk on wine like on any other alcoholic beverage. However, you are better off drinking stronger stuff if your goal is only to get drunk.

There are no known deleterious effects of drinking Red wine. If that were so, no one would be enjoying wine today. On the other hand Red wine is known to prolong healthy life. Many centurions have commented on their daily dose of wine. Red wine is known to be good for the heart. There is less likelihood of heart problems if you consume moderate amount of wine. Red wine also acts as an anti-oxidant. This means that your body cells are protected from the bad effects from ravages of time. It also keeps your skin youthful and face free from wrinkles. You will learn more about the health benefits of Red wine in subsequent chapters.

As mentioned earlier, drinking Red wine is an art. It has to be had deliberately and with time on hand. The joy of having Red wine begins with appreciation of its color and content. Swirling the wine in your glass and smelling the aroma can be a wonderful experience. And then a small little sip can take you to heaven. You must never gulp down wine. It's sacrilegious. You must touch the wine glass to your lips and let the wine softly slip into your mouth. You must feel the warmth of wine going down the throat and enjoy the glorious feeling of it going right down to your stomach.

Wine is the only natural drink which offers a complex array of aromas, fragrances and flavors. Apple juice whether artificially flavored or original, always tastes like apple juice. Milk, whether from cow or a buffalo, still smells like milk. Whisky usually feels like whiskey.

Inhaling a fine wine is like an orchestral experience. You can taste the entire gamut of musical instruments – from the melodious flute to the exuberant saxophone. You can inhale an entire scale of harmonics until your senses are brought to an exhilarating and spectacular finish. A good wine can provide you with an alternate consciousness almost equal to a divine experience.

You might call wine a sensory symphony. The range of smells and fragrances is almost unlimited. Some even call it a sensual experience.

You have to be careful while using words related to wine. The term aroma is used for the smell of a youthful wine. The smell of a mature, more sophisticated wine, which has seen many years in a barrel, is called bouquet. This distinction is easy when you think of the image that goes with each word. When you think of aroma, you tend to think of a single perfume. A bouquet, in contrast, is an intricate arrangement whose fragrance results from the interaction of its multiple constituents.

Body of a wine is determined by the wine's alcohol, glycerin and extract. It's light, moderate or full, and may or may not be in balance with the flavor and other components. The body appears firm with sufficient acidity, or it may be "flabby" when acidity is lacking. It may feel "heavy" from residual sugar, or may feel "harsh," "rough," "coarse," "silky," "velvet," "smooth," or "creamy," depending on its structure.

The tannins in red wines are an important part of wine. It is required to give needed and agreeable astringency to fine wines. It may not seem so pleasing at first sip, but as your wine experience progresses, certain wines will begin to seem flat and dull without it.

You have to mainly observe the clarity and color of Red wine. It should be clear and should not show any cloudiness which is sign of a bad wine. Tasting will reveal this for sure. When a wine is flawed, you will always smell and taste the flaws. On the other hand, a wine with gemlike brilliance is truly a beauty to behold.

Now that you know about the exquisiteness and splendor of the subtle liquid called Red wine, go forth and enjoy. Three cheers to your heath, wealth and happiness.

## How Wine is made?

As the slogan goes "Wine tastes better with age" the taste of wine differs as per the taste of grapes. Wines are cloistered in climate-controlled cellars, aging into works of art. Making of wine has always intrigued and interested people. The grapes are plucked and fermented and bottled. It is very interesting to note that people used to stamp on these grapes to extract the juice. Now machines are doing the job that was done by human legs.

This chart here shows the process of wine making:

Harvesting ⟹ Stemming ⟹ Crushing ⟹ Fermentation ⟹

Pressing ⟹ Finishing ⟹ Bottling

The process –

1. The first step involves removing the leaves and other extraneous material from the grapes.
2. The fruit is then crushed (or pressed) to release the juice and begin the process of maceration. It is important to mention here that stemming and pressing is done soon after the grapes are plucked.
3. For red wines, fermentation is prolonged and occurs simultaneously with alcoholic fermentation. The alcohol generated by yeast action enhances the extraction of anthocyanin and promotes the uptake of tannins from the seeds and skins. The phenolic compounds solubilized give red wines their basic properties of appearance, taste, and flavor. They are also required to give red wines their aging

and mellowing characteristics. In addition, ethanol augments the liberation of aromatic ingredients from the pulp and skins.

4. After partial or complete fermentation, the free-run is allowed to flow away under gravity.
5. Pressing is the last function after which the fine is allowed to rest before it is bottled.
6. Newly bottled wines are normally aged at the winery for several months to years before release. This period permits wines blended shortly before bottling to "harmonize."

Color Matters

The main points to look for in a wine are clarity and color. The wine should be free from a hazy or cloudy look. Haziness is usually a sign of a biological instability or a bacterial or chemical taint, usually from faulty winemaking. Tasting will reveal this for sure. When a wine is flawed, you will always smell and taste the defects. On the other hand, a wine with gemlike brilliance is truly a beauty to behold.

# Types of Glorious Red Wine

Red Wine is available in thousands of varieties, flavors and price. You can have bottle of Chateau Mouton Rothschild costing more than 150,000 USD or you can sip on a simple but delectable glass for as low as $2. Not all costly wines are excellent and nor are the cheaper ones bad. A wine can come with a single aroma or with a bouquet of flavors. Complex wines have layers of flavors and nuances that make it more mysterious and delectable than a simple wine. Some wine experts have described complex wine as "tasting of raspberries with hints of chocolate." That's a bit off the kilter but complex wine cannot be described in any other manner.

What determines the character of a wine: Ideally good wine should be a fine blend of good grape variety, the climate and soil where it is grown, and the winemaker's creative or commercial objective and winemaking skills. That's why you must look at the label of a wine bottle to find out its origin and pedigree. Some winemakers treat wine as a baby and give as much love and care. For some, prize is just a byproduct of their labor of love.

Wine needs appreciation and a sense of subtle taste. A reasonable amount of personal taste also comes into play while separating excellent wine from the good wine. Sometimes or rather usually, understanding the subtlety of wine quality can be confusing and downright confounding. German Rieslings can be way ahead in quality compared to wines made in California from the same grapes. Or Californian Cabernet Sauvignon can outperform Italian Chianti Classico. The only conclusion we can reach, if at all, is that determining quality of wine is a complex task. It is therefore advisable to stick to some simple rules and enjoy your wine rather than spoil the taste with technicalities. At the same time it's best to know what you are drinking to derive maximum pleasure from its consumption.

Now let's look at some classic red wines. We will not be talking about white wine, which are also available in great many varieties.

France is undoubtedly the cradle of wine civilization. It is apt to begin our wine journey from this beautiful country of vineyards and wineries.

## Bordeaux

The name Bordeaux is known well but many don't know the pedigree of this fine wine. Bordeaux is  a industrial city and the wine regions surrounding it in the south west of France. It is by far the largest quality wine region in the world, and the most prolific producer of famous and high quality wines. Bordeaux is the stuff that legends are made of. It's home to such famous names as Chateau Lafite-Rothschild, Chateau Latour and Chateaux Margaux. Thankfully, not all of the region's exports are beyond a normal man's budget. Bordeaux is also known for producing high-quality, highly enjoyable yet affordable wines. Most Bordeaux wines are dry reds.

Red Bordeaux wines are a hearty and robust lot that go well with foods that stand up to them. If red meat is your meal of choice, you've met your match. Red Bordeaux are excellent with steak, rib roasts, venison and lamb. They also go well with game birds, full-flavored, firm fish like salmon, and cheeses like brie, goat cheese, Swiss cheese and parmesan.

## Burgundy

Another popular and well known Red wine is Burgundy. This wine is usually made from grapes grown in Cote d'Or and Cote Chalonnaise. A fine red Burgundy is as different from its Bordeaux as red is from white. It is made from the Pinot Noir grape and is lighter in color. It is medium to full-bodied, and is relatively low in tannin and often silky or velvety on the palate. The aroma is unique to Burgundy with flavors that frequently defy description Flavors often resemble cherries and ripe berries or moss and woodsy mushroom scents. With age, a great Burgundy develops great complexity with subtle nuances of flavor and finesse that can be memorable. A red Burgundy requires from seven to ten years to mature, and great Burgundies can continue to improve for decades.

## Cabernet Sauvignon

Cabernet Sauvignon is the king of the red vini fera. Ideally, Cabernet Sauvignon wines offer great depth of flavor and intensity of color, and develop finesse and breed with aging. Red vinifera grows in all grape regions yielding wines of different quality. In France, Cabernet Sauvignon takes the credit for the lofty reputation of Bordeaux red wines. It's the prime element in many of the finest bottling. In northern Italy, it can yield reasonable likenesses of Bordeaux. Cabernet also grows in many eastern European countries, where it is made into pleasant light wines. Cabernet has taken to California sunshine like a swimmer to a beach. Some of its California bottling are on par with Bordeaux and some have even reached noble quality. Other California Cabernets run the entire quality spectrum. South American countries, particularly Chile and

Argentina, produce Cabernet in vast quantities but with questionable quality.

Cabernet Sauvignon is a versatile vinifera that works well by itself and in the company of other grapes. It's at its best and longest-lived when made with close to 100 percent Cabernet grapes, but it has an affinity for blending with other wines. Cabernet Sauvignon wines are high in tannin and medium- to full-bodied. Their distinctive varietal character is a spicy, bell pepper aroma and flavor with high astringency. Deeply colored wines made from very ripe grapes are often minty with a black currant or cassis character.

**Merlot**

This French variety is grown in many wine regions. As a varietal, it makes wines that are soft and subtle, yet substantial. The finest Merlots possess great depth, complexity and longevity. Merlot is used as a mellowing component Cabernet Sauvignon. In some

In some places in Bordeaux, Merlot is used as an elegant and mellowing component in Cabernet Sauvignon. Merlot is also the star in other places, usually comprising sixty to eighty percent of the blend, and produces complex, velvety, and sometimes quite expensive wines. In California and Italy an increasing number of wineries are producing varietal Merlots, but it is used primarily as a blending agent with the more powerful Cabernet. In California terminology, Merlot is the best supporting actor. Cabernet Sauvignon is still the big box office draw.

Merlot has a distinctive herbaceous aroma quite different from the bell pepper quality of the Cabernet. It is softer in tannins and usually lowers in acidity, producing rounder, fatter, and earlier maturing wine. The very qualities that make Merlot less powerful than Cabernet Sauvignon make it more palatable for some wine drinkers. Don't be intimidated by wine snobs. Merlot is easier to drink by itself and it goes well with lighter foods.

## Pinot Noir

Some call Pinot Noir as one of the noblest of all wine grapes. It is grown throughout the wine world, but success varies due to its sensitivity to soil, climate, and the colonel variant of the vine. This is one temperamental wine variety. In France, Pinot Noir is the principal red grape of the Cote d'Or region of Burgundy, where it produces some of the world's most celebrated and costly wines. With the exception of Blanc de Blanc, it is used as a base for all Champagnes and is admired for body and elegance.

## Zinfandel

Zinfandel is a red variety which is grown only in California, an interesting sort of status. It's originated from Italian grape and therefore has no French lineage. This means it has escaped being compared with French wines. The typical character is berrylike - blackberry or raspberry with a hint of spiciness. Styles vary from light and young to heavy, syrupy and late harvest. Zinfandel reds have a rich, deep color.

## Syrah/Shiraz

Syrah traces its origin back to the days of the Roman and Greek Empires. Its ancestral home is the northern part of the Rhone

Valley, where it is used to make the full-bodied, deeply-colored, powerful, long-lived wines. In Australia, where it's known as the Shiraz or Hermitage grape, it yields potent wines that are often blended with Cabernet. The Syrah is also responsible for South Africa's finest red wines. This is one grape variety where California is lagging behind.

Syrah's firm and full-bodied wines have aromas and flavors that suggest roasted peppers, a la Cabernet Sauvignon, smoked meat, tar, and even burnt rubber. Wonder who drinks these wines, but don't be surprised if there are many who find this exotic. Some of the Australian varieties are softer, less full-bodied, and more berrylike than the archetype Syrah.

## Napa Valley wines – US equivalent of fine French wine

American wine is considered below par by many but the truth is that wines made out of grapes from Napa valley can equal or even surpass many noble wines from France. Napa Valley Cabernet Sauvignon ranks among California's best when made to be the best. Those made from grapes grown from north of Yountville, a cool area south of St. Helena, generally qualify in the mid- or super-premium range. A select few from sites in Rutherford, Oakville, and the Stags Leap district can achieve noble status. Well-made Napa Cabernets offer a berryish, herbal aroma, fairly full body, ample tannins and some warmth. The super-premiums have a riper character, reminiscent of cassis, dried sage, and black currants, that often develops a cedary "cigar-box" characteristic with bottle aging. The best of these will benefit from aging for a decade or more.

Merlot is fast gaining in stature and popularity. It's easier to enjoy since its tannins are less harsh and less astringent than Cabernet. Napa has the edge on quality Merlots. The best are very ripe and herbaceous in aroma and flavor. They have a round, soft, and voluptuous character, and you'll frequently notice a somewhat sweet finish.

Zinfandel thrives in Napa Valley when grown on hillside sites and allowed to ripen to high sugar levels. It does less well on the valley floor. Super-premium Zinfandels come from hillsides or very old vineyards. Zinfandel reigns in the Calistoga region, the area's warmest sub-region.

Most Napa Valley Zinfandels are berry-like, medium-bodied, with moderate tannins and a tart finish. That's red Zinfandel we're talking about. The blush wine, White Zinfandel, has recently soared to popularity. It's a light, sweet and fruity wine, good for summer and leisurely drinking.

Bordeaux styled blended wines have appeared in greater numbers during the past decade. The reds are usually made from red Bordeaux varieties (Cabernet Sauvignon, Cabernet Franc, Merlot, and sometimes Malbec and Petit Verdot).

Most American wines bear varietal names. You've probably noticed that California wines are labeled Chardonnay or Cabernet Sauvignon, while their French equivalents are called Burgundy or Bordeaux. Most European wines are named for the wine region instead of the grape, although this is starting to change as winemakers capitalize on the power of marketing varietal names.

# Red wine and weight loss

Obesity is an issue that is plaguing our society for the last two decades. Every second child is overweight and obese due to which several other complications develop. Thousands of websites talk about weight loss, diet, fitness and nutrition. But no one has mentioned that red wine can actually help you to shed weight. Yes! Red wine can help you with weight loss. That doesn't mean you drink a bottle a day; you just need to have a glass or two daily to help your body shed the excess fat. Drinking red wine in moderation has benefits of weight reduction. A glass or two of red wine has been shown to cut cravings, appetite, and help to make you feel more relaxed, which means less eating and an earlier bedtime, it can also lower your blood pressure. Instead of wasting money trying out diets that promise weight loss but nothing happens, simply drink a glass or two of red wine and see the magic happen.

### *Fights urge to gorge on sweets*

After dinner when you get the urge to gorge on sweet, drinking a glass of red wine will help you to relax and the urge is curbed.

Research shows that resveratrol, an ingredient found in the skin of grapes, berries and red wine can help turn flab into calorie-burning 'brown' fat. Scientist/ researcher Professor Min Du, from Washington State University, US says that Polyphenols that are available in fruits enhances the oxidation of dietary fats so that the body won't get over loaded. They burn the fat as heat there by helping the body to maintain balance thereby preventing obesity and metabolic dysfunction. It also slows the growth of fat cells and formation of new fat cells in the liver.

Grapes contain more polyphenol than other fruits. Grapes are grown in weather conditions that help to keep the fruit from adding heat to the body. In fact several ailments like migraine can be cured with the help of grapes. The colorless juice of red grapes stays in contact with the dark grape skins during fermentation and absorbs the skins' color. Along with color, the grape skins give the wine *tannin,* a substance that's an important part of the way a red wine tastes. Fruits like raspberries, blue berries, strawberries, apples and grapes are rich in these compounds and this in turn helps in losing weight. So you could argue that you could just eat a handful of red grapes and gain the same benefits as a glass of merlot, but a little buzz puts the mind at ease, and adds several other bonuses.

### Contains low fat

Belly fat, or visceral fat, is the most dangerous type of fat. This deadly fat wraps around the organs deep in your abdomen, spiking your risk for diabetes, heart disease, stroke and metabolic syndrome. You can't see or pinch visceral fat, and it's often associated with a large waist. Ditch it with a glass of red wine everyday and you'll not only save your health, you'll also lose weight and trim your waistline.

Many weight loss experts suggest that red wine should be taken along with fruits and vegetables diet for eliminating refined carbohydrates. It is found that a glass of red wine every night increased the levels of the 'good' cholesterol HDL. Its anti- oxidant qualities make it more desirable than white wine. Intake of red wine can convert white fat into beige fat which burns lipids off as heat, helping to keep the body in balance and avoid fatness and metabolic dysfunction.

Dark colored Muscadine grapes that is found in many red wine labels contains a chemical known as ellagic acid. This acid slows the growth of existing fat cells and formation of new ones so that body burns fat faster. This chemical also boosts metabolism of fatty acids in liver cells that improves liver function. Red wine should be taken in moderation. Excess or over dose will only harm your body not yielding any results for weight loss.

Your digestive tract houses a wide variety of bacteria, some good and some bad. Decreases in good bacteria and/or increases in bad bacteria have been linked to a growing list of health issues, including weight gain, type 2 diabetes, and inflammatory bowel disease. Red wine can help shift the types of bacteria in your digestive track so there's more of the good kind, making you healthier and potentially leaner. It is found that a compound in *red wine* can actually block the growth of fat cells.

Red wine contains dietary flavonoid supplements that help to burn the fat and lose weight. It also induces good sleep. Often people binge when they're agitated. And agitation occurs when you've not had good sleep. So a glass or two of red wine daily before bed time acts as a soothing agent to frayed nerves and relaxes the body and mind. This in turn leads to good sleep.

Once you feel refreshed after a good night's sleep you feel energetic the next morning that automatically leads to think positive. So your workout regimen and diet can be performed with enthusiasm. It is important to mention here that drinking red wine alone cannot help you to lose weight. Combine it with a good work out or exercise along with diet. You can see startling results in a month's time.

Wine contains small quantities of several vitamins notably the B vitamins, such as B1 (thiamine), B2 (riboflavin), and B12 (cobalamin). However, wine is virtually devoid of vitamins A, C, D, and K. Red wine consumption helps in nutrient intake.

### Recipe for weight loss

The ideal diet for weight loss is:

*Scrambled eggs for breakfast,*

*Chicken salad for lunch and*

*Chili con carne without rice for dinner,*

*Accompanied by a glass of good quality red wine.*

Have this diet menu for two weeks and you'll see that your waist has shed its extra weight. You'll feel light and your clothes may also seem to hang on you. A glass of red wine makes your dinner seem special and helps to relax the mind and also aid in weight reduction. Wine also has a psycho logic effect on digestion. The association of wine with refined eating promotes slower food consumption, permitting biofeedback mechanisms to induce satiety and regulate food intake. This automatically leads to weight loss.

## Health benefits of red wine

The use of wine as a medicine, or as a carrier for medications, has a long history. It goes back at least to the ancient Egyptians (Lucia, 1963). Ancient Greek and Roman society used wine extensively in herbal medicines.

Making red wine is a process that is very meticulous by nature. Harvesting red wine grapes is the first and most crucial part of making red wine. This is because red wine grapes need to grown at the right time in a particular time cycle so that they will contain right balance of acids and sugar in them – this will give us the right amount of alcoholic content that we want to achieve in the wine.

Helps in Anti Aging - Scientists have found that red wines have higher levels of polyphenols, antioxidants and in general, the darker the wine, the higher the antioxidant content - in tests, cabernet sauvignon grapes were shown to contain the most polyphenols. The wines grown in milder regions such as Bordeaux,

Burgundy, Rioja and California's Napa Valley may have higher antioxidant levels than wines from hot regions such as Languedoc in France and Southern Italy. This helps the body to live longer and aids anti aging. Some of the longest living people on earth drink red wine in moderation daily.

Red wine helps us to digest our food in a better manner. If you will have it with your food, you will be aiding your body to digest your food as it can break up food effectively. And since it is good for food digestion, it will benefit anyone who wants to lose weight. Recent studies have shown that it contains resveratrol that may allow us to live longer. Finally it creates a calming effect on our body; this in turn helps us to sleep better. If you suffer from insomnia, you will definitely notice a positive change in your sleeping problems once you start consuming red wine. But you need to remember that all benefits of red wine are possible only if you drink it in moderation. Don't try to get drunk when you want to consume it. Red wine can help you live longer.

Good for Skin – There are many facials and massages done at spa and salons with grapes. This fruit facial helps to rejuvenate the skin. The wonderful body massage with grape pulp enters through the pores of the skin to refresh the skin as well as help in blood circulation. It makes the person feel fresh and invigorated. Often women develop crow feet near the eyes and wrinkles on the face. Instead of using Botox or other injectibles it is better to get a grape fruit massage. Even red wine can be mixed to a massage cream and used as a substitute for fresh grapes. It adds instant glow to the face and body. This massage or facial with red wine is known as Vinotherapy.

The antioxidant properties present in red wine help in getting the toxins out of the skin. Wine facials are also great for skin tightening.

- **Do It Yourself Facials**

For sensitive skin add red wine along with rose water and a massage cream. The fragrance of rose water and red wine will make the person feel rejuvenated.

For dry skin add red wine along with almond paste and massage cream. Gently rub the mixture all over the face and massage for a good ten minutes. Later put on a face pack of almonds. You can do this at home.

For oily skin add red wine with aloe vera to the massage cream. Red wine has de-stressing properties and helps you to relax. At the same time it can be used as a beauty product also.

Aids in Digestion - Wine has several direct and indirect effects on food digestion. The phenolic and alcohol contents of wine activate the release of saliva. In addition, wine promotes the release of gastrin as well as gastric juices. Succinic acid is the principal wine ingredient activating the release of gastric juices. It does not, however, activate gastrin release. The substance(s) involved in stimulating gastrin secretion are unknown. Wine also significantly delays gastric emptying, both on an empty stomach or when consumed with food. The latter favors digestion by extending acid hydrolysis. It also promotes inactivation of pathogenic food contaminants. In addition, wine slows plasma glucose uptake, independent of any insulin response. Furthermore, at the levels found in most table wines, ethanol activates the release of bile in the intestines. Wine acids and aromatics also induce the same effects. In contrast, the high alcohol content of distilled beverages can suppress digestive juice flow the release of bile, and induce stomach spasms.

Despite the general beneficial effects of alcohol on digestion, the phenolic content of red wine may retard digestion. For example, tannins and phenolic acids interfere with the action of certain digestive enzymes, such as α-amylase, lipase and trypsin. Digestion may be further delayed by polymerization between tannins and food proteins. Although potentially delaying digestion in the small intestine, it continues in the colon. In contrast, some phenolics, such as quercetin, resveratrol, catechin, and epigallocatechin gallate, promote pepsin-activated protein breakdown.

## Reduces Migraine Attacks – To get rid of migraine you first need to know why and when it occurs. When a person is weak physically and is under lot of stress headache normally occurs. Migraine is a type of headache that starts at the base of the neck and the pain travels all around the head. The pounding at the middle of the head is unbearable. A pain killer along with adequate rest in a dark room can help you to ease the ache. Giddiness and nausea are also side effects of migraine.

There are two main reasons for migraine to occur.

1. Acidity due to not eating for long intervals of time. This can even lead to constipation that causes migraine.
2. Acute stress and tension.

If you eat regularly and at regular intervals then you can keep migraine away. Munching on a handful of red and black grapes along with yoghurt daily at breakfast can help you top keep migraine away. If you're not a fruit lover then substitute it with red wine. Drink two glasses of red wine daily before bed time and see the miracle of getting rid of migraine. Since red wine soothes frayed nerves you relax and sleep well. Having a good bowel movement is essential. Drinking red wine ensures that you can have a good bowel movement to rid of acidity. This ensures you enjoy a headache free life.

Usually a drunken person always has a hangover with a headache the next morning. But in the case of drinking red wine in moderation it rids you of hangover and headache. So you see drinking red wine in moderation will help you to remain fit and healthy.

Cardio Vascular Health – Increased awareness of the risks of lifestyle ailments like high blood pressure, coronary arterial diseases (CAD) etc have made "high cholesterol levels" a familiar phrase. Cholesterol is a lipid also known as fat required by the body to build cell membranes and to produce certain essential hormones. It is available in the body mostly from diet or is endogenous (i.e. synthesized within the body) when availability of the former is inadequate. The liver combines the cholesterol with certain proteins to produce a substance called a lipoprotein, which transports the lipid to the cells through the bloodstream.

Two types of lipoproteins are produced — the 'low density lipoprotein' (LDL) and the 'high density lipoprotein' (HDL). The LDL cholesterol is often referred to as 'bad' cholesterol since excessive concentration of LDL in the blood results in fat deposits (plaque) on the artery walls. This leads to narrowing of arteries (*atherosclerosis*) increasing blood pressure and chances of heart attacks or strokes. The HDL cholesterol, on the other hand, is called 'good' cholesterol as it is believed to 'clean up' arteries. The exact causes and effects of the 'clean-up' process is not, as yet, well understood. It is believed that the HDL molecules are able to pick up cholesterol from the cells they interact with. These are transported back to the liver for reuse or excretion. Thus, a high LDL/HDL ratio is a risk factor for atherosclerosis while the opposite i.e. a low LDL level with higher HDL level (low LDL/HDL ratio) is desirable.

Red wine helps us to protect our hearts. It contains flavanoids that are originally a part of grape skin that then becomes a part of wine when it is being prepared. Flavanoids help us in avoiding bad cholesterol and are very useful as they prevent clotting of blood. Drinking a glass of red wine every night increases levels of good cholesterol HDL while helping reduce the bad, LDL. According to researchers and data obtained, it also helps to lower the risk of heart attack and stroke.

'Tannins' that is present in red wine is what gives the red color to it. Tannins contain procyanidins, known for protecting against heart disease. Resveratrol also helps to remove chemicals responsible for causing blood clots, which is the primary cause of heart attacks. Daily consumption of red wine cuts blood clot and related stroke rates by 50%.

**Protects against Cancer** - Red wine contains a fair amount of Vitamin B and potassium besides also containing sodium in small quantities. Resveratrol that is present in grapes is a powerful antioxidant that can help prevent a variety of different cancers. All these substances are important in helping us to remain healthy. It is also very handy as it is an effective aid for fighting against cancer. The active antioxidant in red wine known as quercetin can kill cancer cells and also helps induce natural cell death in certain types of cancers, most often colon cancer.

**Reduces memory loss** – Red wine has been useful for good health especially for heart health. Now it has also been found that it can actually aid in reducing memory loss. A researcher from Texas A&M has proved that antioxidant present in red wine has positive effects on the brain's hippocampus, which is the part responsible for functions such as mood, learning and memory. Resveratrol has the ability to reduce memory degeneration and help people who're suffering from Alzheimer's and Dementia. It's also great for heart health and preventing Alzheimer's, as it helps prevent cell damage.

The study was conducted on rats and it showed that development of neurons doubled in rats that were treated with resveratrol. Even the blood flow in these rats was better and improved than the ones who weren't given. There was also reduction in inflammation.

## Lowers Blood Sugar in Type II diabetes –

Various studies have shown that diabetes in addition to being hereditary is a lifestyle disease. As more people lead a sedentary life, diabetes is likely to take its toll more often than not. You will generally not see a farmhand suffering from diabetes; while on the other hand, obese desk jobbers contact diabetes easily. The incidence of diabetes has increased manifold because of the easy availability of sugar. Our bodies have never been exposed to such a large amount of sugar, ever before human evolutionary history. Sugar in the form of honey was a rare treat. Due to this our pancreas has been designed to secrete less quantity of insulin. Now when our bodies are exposed to very high level of sugary substances, our pancreas is unable to cater to the additional load.

Type 2 diabetes appears to result when body cells do not respond properly to the presence of insulin. Dietary restrictions are usually recommended in case of diabetes. Unfortunately, the nature of the disease is such that it leads to craving for food. As a person becomes more insulin resistant, his body craves for glucose which in turn leads to high level of sugar. The chain reaction continues to increase the blood sugar level to the detriment of the patient.

Breaking this chain reaction is the first step towards controlling blood glucose levels in diabetic patients.

One of the measures recommended for diabetic patients is therefore to consume more fiber. Fiber can be found in plenty in vegetables and fruits. Some fruits may be contra indicative because of their glucose content. When a person suffering from diabetes feels hungry, vegetable intake may assist in filling the stomach and reduce the craving for more food. Since most of the fiber simply goes through the digestive track without being digested, there is almost no effect on the blood glucose levels.

Since red wine helps in weight loss, it also reduces blood pressure, helps to burn fat from the liver; automatically it helps to reduce blood sugar. Wine consumption has been shown to attenuate insulin resistance in type 2 diabetes. Neil Shay, a biochemist from Oregan State University found that red wine boosted the metabolism of fatty acids in liver cells. "If we could develop a dietary strategy for reducing the harmful accumulation of fat in the liver, using common foods like grapes," Shay says, "that would be good news".

It could help improve type 2 diabetes because it boosts glucose metabolism. This is the process by which simple sugar found in many foods are processed and used to produce energy.

## Strengthens Immune system – Resveratrol is a polyphenol that could be responsible for wine's longevity benefits, researchers believe any diet rich in polyphenols is beneficial, they are known for protecting against chronic disease. Half a glass of wine provides the

benefits of sleep induction, without causing agitation and sleep apnea – often associated with greater alcohol consumption. The effect on sleep may arise from alcohol facilitating the transmission of inhibitory γ-aminobutyric acid (GABA), while suppressing the action of excitatory glutamate receptors (Haddad, 2004). GABA and glutamate are estimated to be involved in about 80% of neuronal circuitry in the brain.

Intake of red wine has reduced hormonal secretion especially vasopressin. Wine is also active against several viruses like herpes simplex virus, poliovirus, hepatitis A virus, as well as rhinoviruses and coronaviruses. The effect on the latter two groups appears reflected in the reduced incidence of common cold in moderate alcohol consumers particularly those drinking red wines. If you have to gargle, port wine is certainly one of the more pleasant options available.

## Reduce calories – One of the chemicals found in the grapes dramatically slowed the growth of fat cells and formation of new ones. It also boosted the metabolism of fatty acids in liver cells.

The low sodium/high potassium content of wine makes it one of the more effective sources of potassium for individuals on diuretics. Although wine contains soluble dietary fiber, especially red wines. It is insufficient to contribute significantly to the daily recommended fiber content in the human diet.

## Helps to see (eye health) with clarity - As you age eye health takes precedence over others. With age the progressive degeneration of the central region of the retina (macula) leads to

blurred or distorted vision. As a consequence it results in local atherosclerosis that deprives the retina of oxygen and nutrients. It is the leading cause of blindness in adults over the age of 65. A similar relationship has been found for cataract development. In both situations, wine antioxidants are suspected to be the active protective agent. Drinking wine may help to reduce the degeneration of retina thereby aiding you to see with clarity.

Even osteoporosis, gout and bone related diseases can be protected by just drinking a glass of wine.

## Osteoporosis – Basically women post menopause develop osteoporosis. It is here that wine can help to prevent bone degeneration and maintain retention in women. The phytoestrogen effects of phenolics, such as resveratrol help the bone to remain strong and protect it from erosion.

## Gout – This is actually the swelling of joints. Gout is often associated with reduced excretion of uric acid in the kidneys. Though alcohol consumption can affect the joints it has not been found about red wine. It actually enhances and favors uric acid absorption by the kidneys.

## Arthritis - Arthritis is a bone related issue. Your body starts to ache and the pain can be quite debilitating. The drugs used to treat arthritis have the tendency to affect the stomach lining. Moderate intake of wine may accrue from its mildly diuretic and muscle-relaxant properties. The diuretic action of wine can help reduce water retention and minimize joint swelling. Wine can also directly

reduce muscle spasms and the stiffness associated with arthritis. The anti-inflammatory influences of wine phenolics, notably resveratrol, may also play a role in diminishing the suffering associated with arthritis.

Kidney Stones – Usually you're advised to drink plenty of water to get rid of kidney stones. Drinking water has long been associated with reducing the development of kidney stones. Increased urine production helps prevent the crystallization of calcium oxalate in the kidneys. What is new is the observation that wine consumption reduces the production of these painful and dangerous inclusions. Just like water red wine also helps to flush out the toxins there by keeping the kidneys in optimum health. Instead of drinking water you can drink a glass or two of red wine at night so that you have good digestion and bowel movements there by reducing the risk of kidney stones.

Wine & medication - If you're on any medication then consult your doctor before taking red wine. Even small consumption of alcohol can cause contra indications like loss of muscle control leading to serious damages. In combination with certain anti-diabetic agents, such as tolbutamide and chlorpropamide, alcohol can cause dizziness, hot flushes, and nausea. Mild reactions may occur with a wide range of other medications, such as sulfanilamide, isoniazid and aminopyrine. It is clear that excessive alcohol consumption, both acute and chronic, can have devastating effects on physical and mental wellbeing. Whereas if you consume in moderation then you can lead a stress free life rid of diseases and risks.

There are umpteen health benefits for red wine consumption. So, raise a toast of cheers to your health!

## Red wine intake helps to prevent dental problems

Regular intake of red wine and grape juice can help to remove bacteria from the teeth. These bacteria produce acid which damages the teeth over time leading to teeth decay. Drinking red wine can protect against cavities. Almost 60% of the world population is affected by some kind of teeth problem. Be it cavities, gum diseases or tooth loss the problem is severe in all the countries around the world.

The problem starts when certain bacteria in the mouth get together and form biofilms, which are a bunch of bacteria that are difficult to kill. They form plaque and produce acid, which damages the teeth. Though Brushing, fluoride in toothpaste and water and other methods can help to get rid of bacterial plaques, the effects are limited.

Research has previously suggested that grape seed extract and wine can slow the growth of bacteria and prevent formation of cavities. Hundreds of microbial species exist within the human mouth simultaneously. Because the teeth are "non-shedding surfaces," microorganisms are able to stick to them for long periods of time, which can lead to the formation of biofilms and dental plaque. Forming a symbiotic relationship within dental plaque, bacteria such as streptococci or lactobacilli are able to produce organic acids in high levels following the fermentation of dietary sugars. These acids demineralize the surface of the teeth, eventually leading to periodontal disease or tooth loss.

The anti-oxidant properties of polyphenols could be useful in the prevention and treatment of inflammatory gum disease. Chemicals in red wine can stop bacteria sticking to extracted teeth in a petri dish, but this does not necessarily mean that drinking red wine will reduce the risk of cavities. It is possible that other components in the wine, such as sugar and acids, could counteract the effects, so that the wine does not remain in the mouth long enough.

Red wine without alcohol inhibits the growth of certain bacteria found in oral biofilm. They help to prevent caries. The researchers also reported that red wine and de-alcoholized red wine were effective in limiting growth of F. nucleatum and S. oralis. This clearly shows that red wine is good for periodontal issues. Research has also found that, for the main component in the de-alcoholized red wine to have this effect was a group of chemicals called proanthocyanidins. The researchers also showed that de-alcoholised red wine made it more difficult for the bacteria to attach and form a thin layer (a biofilm) on the surface of the extracted human tooth.

Each and every part of our body requires repair and healing from time to time. Oral hygiene is very important as a smile will help you to not only boast your pearly whites but also enhance the beauty of the face and improve/ lift your self esteem. A beautiful smile can attract the opposite sex to you and if bad breath or foul smell emanates it can put the person off you. So it is important to maintain oral hygiene not only to keep away from brain related diseases but also to get lead an active social life.

Instead of wasting your time and money in dental clinics simply open a bottle of red wine and drink a couple of glasses daily, to keep your pearly whites in optimum health and boast a magnificent smile that can make you alluring to others. Just as Mother Theresa said once "Peace begins with a smile", so here's raising a toast to a – Beautiful You!

## How to use red wine in cooking?

Wine always reminds us of exotic food at a beautiful restaurant with an attractive companion, candle lights glowing and setting the mood for a romantic evening. Be it Champagne or Napa Valley Cabernet Sauvignon the taste of red wine transport you to a different world of happiness and joy. The best chefs in the world swear by this red liquid that adds taste to gourmet food. There are several interesting recopies that can be made with the help of red wine. Since it aids in weight loss, it's all the more important to add red wine in your daily diet.

A long-simmered leg of lamb or beef roast calls for a correspondingly hearty wine, such as a Petite Syrah or a Zinfandel. A lighter dish might call for a less powerful red—think Pinot Noir or Chianti. Get to know Port, Sherry, Madeira, and Marsala. These are among the best wines good cooks can have on hand.

You can make amazing sauces and stews with the help of red wine. You can also add them to fruit salad or a vegetable salad giving it an extra richness. Red wine can also be used in spaghetti with walnuts and parsley.

**Here's the recipe:**

Ingredients:

One packet spaghetti

Virgin olive oil

Red Wine

Chopped Parsley

Red Pepper

Garlic cloves

Roasted Almonds

Walnuts

Cheese


Method:

Boil three cups of water along with one cup of red wine. Add spaghetti to the boiling water and cook for ten to fifteen minutes. Once the spaghetti is cooked, drain the water and let it to cool. Meanwhile take a pan and heat virgin olive oil. Add parsley, garlic and red pepper. Sauté for five minutes before adding roasted almonds and walnuts that are coarsely crushed. Add spaghetti to this mixture and pour red wine over it. Grate cheese on top of the spaghetti. Add salt to taste.

Dressing:

Remove the spaghetti in a dish and sprinkle cheese and almonds over it. Decorate with a parsley leaf and walnuts.

You can use the same method with noodles and pasta also. In case you like your spaghetti spicy add bell pepper and a couple of green chilies.

Since red wine is used in cooking it'll help you to lose weight. Instead of using fatty oils or weight inducing wines you can supplement it with red wine.

### Cook lamb and meat in red wine

Cooking with red wine makes your meal light and easy to digest. While cooking lamb or meat, slow cook it in red wine and the meat will taste succulent. Add lime juice to it with a dash of pepper and your meat is ready to be gorged on. The flavor of red wine with pepper brings out the fragrance and aroma of the meat. Lime juice adds the citrus taste complementing the red wine.

Red wine blends beautifully with risotto, fish and meat. The richness of red wine adds a dash of expensive taste to the dish. Also it's not very expensive. At $25 you can get a bottle of red wine that can help you to cook gourmet food. And not to forget that it'll help in digestion and aids weight loss. Cook your food with red wine and see yourself losing weight and slipping back into your skinny jeans that you bought ten years ago.

# Conclusion

Now that you've read the book you can drink a glass or two daily to lose weight and keep healthy. Drinking red wine and using it in cooking can help you with a whole lot of health benefits that have been discussed in this book. This book is a sincere attempt to get you all the necessary information that a person should know before you drink a bottle of your favorite Cabernet Sauvignon. So drink red wine and lose weight dramatically. Combined with dieting and regular exercise soon you'll be slipping into your skinny pair of jeans that you wore ten years ago.

So what are you waiting for?

Go ahead raise a toast and say CHEERS to your favorite red wine to a slimmer you!